YOUR BODY WILL THANK YOU

Why a Low-Calorie Diet is Good for Healthy Living

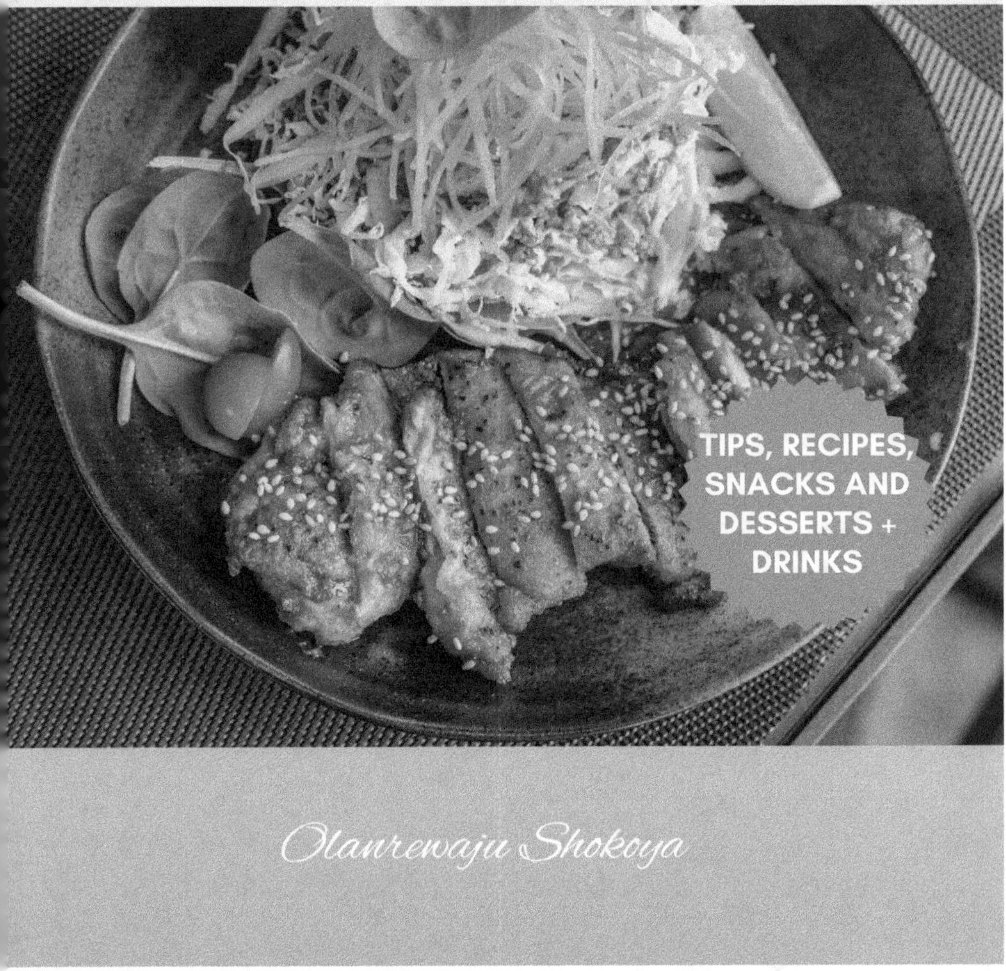

TIPS, RECIPES, SNACKS AND DESSERTS + DRINKS

Olanrewaju Shokoya

Author's detail: Shokoya O.M, Importance of Healthy Living: Benefits c
a Low-Calorie Diet, Email: Olanshoksconsulting@gmail.com. June 202
Pretoria, South Africa.

CONTENT

Introduction
- Importance of Healthy Living
- Benefits of a Low-Calorie Diet

Chapter 1: Understanding Calories
- What Are Calories?
- Caloric Needs and How to Calculate Them
- Myths and Facts About Calories

Chapter 2: Tips for Healthy Living
- Balanced Diet Essentials
- Importance of Hydration
- Regular Exercise
- Quality Sleep
- Mindful Eating

Chapter 3: Meal Planning
- How to Create a Low-Calorie Meal Plan
- Grocery Shopping Tips
- Sample Weekly Meal Plans

Chapter 4: Breakfast Recipes
- Smoothie Bowls
- Overnight Oats
- Low-Calorie Pancakes
- Healthy Breakfast Burritos

Introduction

Welcome to a culinary journey that celebrates the art of healthy living through delicious, low-calorie cuisine. In today's fast-paced world, finding balance between nutrition and flavour can often feel like a daunting task. However, this cookbook is here to show you that nourishing your body with wholesome, low-calorie meals can be both fulfilling and enjoyable.

Embracing the Benefits of a Low-Calorie Diet

Incorporating a low-calorie diet into your lifestyle offers numerous benefits beyond weight management. It can enhance your overall well-being by reducing the risk of chronic diseases, improving digestion, boosting energy levels, and supporting mental clarity. By focusing on nutrient-dense ingredients and mindful eating, you'll not only feel better physically but also cultivate a deeper connection to the food you consume.

Discovering Delicious and Nutritious Recipes

Within these pages, you'll find a collection of recipes meticulously crafted to tantalize your taste buds while supporting your health goals. From vibrant salads and hearty soups to satisfying main dishes and guilt-free desserts, each recipe is designed to showcase the natural flavours of fresh, wholesome ingredients. Whether you're a seasoned home cook or just beginning your culinary journey, there's something here to inspire and delight every palate.

A Guide to Sustainable Eating Habits

Beyond the recipes themselves, this cookbook serves as a guide to cultivating sustainable eating habits that you can maintain for life. You'll learn how to navigate grocery aisles, make informed food choices, and incorporate variety into your meals without sacrificing taste or nutritional value. By embracing these principles, you'll not only transform the way you eat but also the way you live.

Your Journey Starts Here.

So, embark on this journey with an open mind and a willingness to explore the endless possibilities of healthy, low-calorie cooking. Let this cookbook be your companion in creating meals that nourish both body and soul. Here's to vibrant health, culinary creativity, and savouring every delicious moment along the way.

Shokoya O.M

Chapter 1: Understanding Calories

What Are Calories?

Calories are units of energy that our bodies use to function. Everything we do, from breathing and thinking to walking and exercising, requires energy. This energy comes from the food and drinks we consume. The amount of energy provided by food is measured in calories.

Caloric Needs and How to Calculate Them

Each person's caloric needs are different and depend on various factors such as age, gender, weight, height, and activity level. Knowing your daily caloric needs is essential for maintaining a healthy weight and supporting overall well-being.

Basal Metabolic Rate (BMR)

Your Basal Metabolic Rate (BMR) is the number of calories your body needs to perform basic life-sustaining functions, such as breathing, circulation, and cell production, while at rest. You can calculate your BMR using the following formulas:

• **For Women**: BMR=655+(9.6×weight in kg) +(1.8×height in cm)
-(4.7×age in years) BMR = 655 + (9.6 \times \text {weight in kg}) + (1.8
\times \text {height in cm}) – (4.7 \times \text {age in years})
BMR=655+(9.6×weight in kg) + (1.8×height in cm) -(4.7×age in years)

• **For Men**: BMR=66+(13.7×weight in kg) +(5×height in cm) -(6.8×age in
years) BMR = 66 + (13.7 \times \text {weight in kg}) + (5 \times \text
{height in cm}) – (6.8 \times \text {age in years}) BMR=66+(13.7×weight
in kg) +(5×height in cm) -(6.8×age in years)

Total Daily Energy Expenditure (TDEE)

Your Total Daily Energy Expenditure (TDEE) is the total number of
calories you need in a day, considering your activity level. To calculate
your TDEE, multiply your BMR by an activity factor:

• Sedentary (little or no exercise): BMR × 1.2
• Lightly active (light exercise/sports 1-3 days/week): BMR × 1.375
• Moderately active (moderate exercise/sports 3-5 days/week): BMR ×
1.55
• Very active (hard exercise/sports 6-7 days a week): BMR × 1.725
• Super active (very hard exercise/sports & a physical job): BMR × 1.9
For example, if your BMR is 1500 calories and you are lightly active,
your TDEE would be: TDEE=1500×1.375=2062.5 calories/dayTDEE =
1500 \times 1.375 = 2062.5 \text{calories/day}
TDEE=1500×1.375=2062.5 calories/day

Myths and Facts About Calories

There are many misconceptions about calories and dieting. Here are some common myths and the facts that debunk them:

Myth 1: All Calories Are Equal Fact: While a calorie is a unit of energy, the source of those calories matters. Nutrient-dense foods, like fruits, vegetables, and whole grains, provide more than just calories – they offer vitamins, minerals, and fibre. Empty calories from sugary drinks and processed foods provide energy but little nutritional value.

Myth 2: Cutting More Calories is Always Better Fact: Severely restricting calories can be harmful to your health. It can slow down your metabolism, lead to nutrient deficiencies, and cause muscle loss. It's important to create a moderate calorie deficit to lose weight safely and sustainably.

Myth 3: Eating Late at Night Causes Weight Gain Fact: Weight gain occurs when you consume more calories than you burn, regardless of the time of day you eat. However, late-night snacking can lead to consuming excess calories, especially if you're eating out of habit rather than hunger.

Myth 4: You Must Count Calories to Lose Weight Fact: While counting calories can be an effective tool for weight loss, it's not the only approach. Focusing on whole, unprocessed foods, listening to your body's hunger and fullness cues, and maintaining a balanced diet can also help you achieve and maintain a healthy weight.

Myth 5: Low-Calorie Diets are Always Healthy Fact: Not all low-calorie diets are nutritious. It's crucial to ensure that your diet is balanced and includes a variety of nutrients. Aim for a diet rich in fruits, vegetables, lean proteins, whole grains, and healthy fats to support overall health. Understanding calories and their role in your diet is the first step towards making informed decisions about your food choices. By learning how to calculate your caloric needs and debunking common myths, you can set a solid foundation for a healthy lifestyle.

Chapter 2: Tips for Healthy Living

Balanced Diet Essentials

A balanced diet is crucial for maintaining good health and providing your body with the nutrients it needs to function correctly. Here are the key components of a balanced diet:

• **Fruits and Vegetables**: Aim to fill half your plate with fruits and vegetables. They are rich in vitamins, minerals, and fibre, and low in calories.

- **Whole Grains**: Choose whole grains like brown rice, quinoa, oats, and whole wheat bread over refined grains. They provide more nutrients and fibre.
- **Lean Proteins:** Include a variety of protein sources such as poultry, fish, beans, lentils, tofu, and nuts. Lean proteins help build and repair tissues.
- **Dairy or Dairy Alternatives:** opt for low-fat or fat-free dairy products, or fortified dairy alternatives like almond or soy milk.
- **Healthy Fats**: Incorporate healthy fats from sources like avocados, olive oil, nuts, and seeds. These fats support brain health and reduce inflammation.

Importance of Hydration

Staying hydrated is essential for overall health. Water plays a vital role in various bodily functions, including digestion, temperature regulation, and nutrient transport. Here are some tips to ensure you stay adequately hydrated:

- **Drink Plenty of Water:** Aim for at least 8 cups (64 ounces) of water a day. This amount can vary depending on factors like activity level, climate, and individual needs.
- **Monitor Your Urine**: A good indicator of hydration is the colour of your urine. Light yellow or clear urine usually means you are well-hydrated.
- **Eat Hydrating Foods**: Incorporate water-rich foods into your diet, such as cucumbers, watermelon, strawberries, and lettuce.
- **Limit Sugary Drinks**: Reduce your intake of sugary beverages like soda and juice, which can contribute to dehydration.

Regular Exercise

Exercise is a cornerstone of a healthy lifestyle. It helps maintain a healthy weight, improves cardiovascular health, and boosts mood and energy levels. Here are some tips to incorporate regular exercise into your routine:

Find an Activity You Enjoy: Choose exercises that you find enjoyable, whether it's walking, cycling, dancing, or swimming. This increases the likelihood that you will stick with it.

- **Set Realistic Goals**: Start with achievable goals and gradually increase the intensity and duration of your workouts. Aim for at least 150 minutes of moderate aerobic activity or 75 minutes of vigorous activity each week.
- **Incorporate Strength Training**: Include strength training exercises at least twice a week. This can involve lifting weights, using resistance bands, or bodyweight exercises like push-ups and squats.
- **Stay Active Throughout the Day**: Look for opportunities to move more during your daily routine. Take the stairs, walk or bike instead of driving, and stand up and stretch regularly if you have a sedentary job.

Quality Sleep

Quality sleep is essential for physical and mental health. Poor sleep can lead to various health issues, including weight gain, weakened immunity, and reduced cognitive function. Here are some tips for better sleep:

- **Establish a Routine**: Go to bed and wake up at the same time every day, even on weekends. This helps regulate your body's internal clock.
- **Create a Relaxing Environment**: Make your bedroom conducive to sleep by keeping it cool, dark, and quiet. Consider using blackout curtains, earplugs, or a white noise machine.
- **Limit Screen Time Before Bed**: Avoid screens from TVs, computers, and smartphones at least an hour before bedtime. The blue light emitted by these devices can interfere with your sleep cycle.
- **Avoid Stimulants**: Limit caffeine and nicotine intake, especially in the afternoon and evening. These substances can disrupt your sleep.

Mindful Eating

Mindful eating involves paying full attention to the experience of eating and enjoying your food without distractions. It can help you develop a healthier relationship with food and improve digestion.

Here are some tips for practicing mindful eating:
Eat Slowly: Take your time to chew and savour each bite. This allows your body to register feelings of fullness and prevents overeating.

- **Listen to Your Body**: Pay attention to hunger and fullness cues. Eat when you're hungry and stop when you're satisfied, not when you're stuffed.
- **Eliminate Distractions:** Avoid eating while watching TV, working, or using your phone. Focus on your meal and the experience of eating.
- **Appreciate Your Food**: Take a moment to appreciate the colours, textures, and flavours of your food. This can enhance your enjoyment and satisfaction.

By incorporating these tips into your daily routine, you can create a foundation for a healthy and balanced lifestyle. Remember, small changes can lead to significant improvements in your overall well-being.

Chapter 3: Meal Planning

How to Create a Low-Calorie Meal Plan

Creating a low-calorie meal plan involves careful planning to ensure you meet your nutritional needs while keeping your calorie intake in check. Here are some steps to help you get started:

1.**Determine Your Caloric Needs**: Use the information from Chapter 1 to calculate your Total Daily Energy Expenditure (TDEE). Aim to create a calorie deficit of 500-1000 calories per day for a healthy weight loss of 1-2 pounds per week.
2.**Plan Balanced Meals**: Ensure each meal includes a mix of lean proteins, healthy fats, and complex carbohydrates. This balance will help keep you full and satisfied.
3.**Incorporate Plenty of Vegetables**: Vegetables are low in calories and high in nutrients. Fill half your plate with a variety of colourful veggies.

.**Choose Whole Foods**: opt for whole, unprocessed foods over
packaged and processed options. Whole foods are generally lower in
calories and higher in nutrients.
.**Watch Portion Sizes**: Be mindful of portion sizes to avoid overeating.
Use measuring cups, a food scale, or visual cues to keep portions in
check.
.**Stay Hydrated**: Drink plenty of water throughout the day.
Sometimes, thirst can be mistaken for hunger.

Grocery Shopping Tips

Effective grocery shopping is key to sticking to your low-calorie meal
plan. Here are some tips to help you make healthier choices:
Make a List: Plan your meals for the week and create a shopping list
based on your meal plan. Stick to the list to avoid impulse purchases.
.**Shop the Perimeter**: The outer aisles of the grocery store typically
contain fresh produce, lean meats, and dairy products. Avoid the inner
aisles where processed and packaged foods are located.
.**Read Labels**: Pay attention to nutrition labels and ingredient lists.
Look for foods that are low in added sugars, sodium, and unhealthy
fats.
.**Buy in Season:** Seasonal fruits and vegetables are often fresher,
more nutritious, and more affordable.
.**Stock Up on Staples**: Keep your pantry stocked with healthy staples
like whole grains, beans, nuts, seeds, and spices. This makes it easier to
prepare healthy meals.

Sample Weekly Meal Plans

Here are two sample weekly meal plans to give you an idea of how to
structure your meals. Each plan includes three meals and two snacks
per day.

Sample Meal Plan 1:

Monday:
  - Breakfast: Greek yogurt with berries and a sprinkle of chia seeds
  - Snack: Apple slices with almond butter
  - Lunch: Quinoa salad with mixed greens, cherry tomatoes, cucumbers,
    and grilled chicken
  - Snack: Carrot sticks with hummus
  - Dinner: Baked salmon with steamed broccoli and brown rice

- **Tuesday:**
o Breakfast: Smoothie made with spinach, banana, frozen berries, and almond milk
o Snack: Handful of mixed nuts
o Lunch: Turkey and avocado wrap with a side of baby carrots
o Snack: Low-fat cottage cheese with pineapple chunks
o Dinner: Stir-fried tofu with bell peppers, snap peas, and quinoa
- **Wednesday:**
o Breakfast: Overnight oats with almond milk, chia seeds, and sliced strawberries
o Snack: Sliced cucumber with tzatziki
o Lunch: Lentil soup with a side salad
o Snack: Sliced bell peppers with guacamole
o Dinner: Grilled chicken breast with roasted sweet potatoes and asparagus
- **Thursday:**
o Breakfast: Scrambled eggs with spinach and tomatoes
o Snack: Orange slices
o Lunch: Mixed greens with chickpeas, cherry tomatoes, cucumbers, and a light vinaigrette
o Snack: Air-popped popcorn
o Dinner: Zucchini noodles with marinara sauce and turkey meatballs
- **Friday:**
o Breakfast: Smoothie bowl with mixed berries, banana, and a sprinkle of granola
o Snack: Celery sticks with peanut butter
o Lunch: Whole grain wrap with hummus, roasted veggies, and spinach
o Snack: Greek yogurt with a drizzle of honey
o Dinner: Baked cod with quinoa and sautéed kale

Sample Meal Plan 2:
- **Saturday:**
o Breakfast: Low-calorie pancakes with fresh blueberries
o Snack: Pear slices with cottage cheese
o Lunch: Spinach and feta stuffed chicken breast with a side of quinoa
o Snack: Cherry tomatoes with mozzarella balls

o Dinner: Veggie stir-fry with tofu and brown rice
• **Sunday:**
o Breakfast: Smoothie with kale, mango, and coconut water
o Snack: Hard-boiled egg
o Lunch: Shrimp salad with mixed greens, avocado, and a light lemon dressing
o Snack: Fresh pineapple chunks
o Dinner: Turkey chili with a side of steamed green beans

By following these steps and using the sample meal plans as a guide, you can create a low-calorie meal plan that suits your preferences and lifestyle. Consistent planning and mindful shopping will help you stay on track and achieve your health goals.

Chapter 4: Breakfast Recipes

Smoothie Bowls

Smoothie bowls are a delicious and visually appealing way to start your day. They are versatile and can be customized with your favourite fruits, nuts, and seeds.

Berry Bliss Smoothie Bowl Ingredients:
- 1 cup frozen mixed berries (strawberries, blueberries, raspberries)
- 1 banana
- 1/2 cup unsweetened almond milk
- 1/4 cup Greek yogurt
- 1 tablespoon chia seeds
- Toppings: sliced strawberries, blueberries, granola, sliced almonds

Instructions:
1. Blend the frozen berries, banana, almond milk, Greek yogurt, and chia seeds until smooth.
2. Pour the smoothie into a bowl.
3. Add your favourite toppings, such as sliced strawberries, blueberries, granola, and sliced almonds.
4. Serve immediately and enjoy!

Green Goddess Smoothie Bowl Ingredients:
- 1 cup spinach
- 1 banana
- 1/2 avocado
- 1/2 cup unsweetened almond milk
- 1 tablespoon flax seeds
- Toppings: kiwi slices, shredded coconut, pumpkin seeds

Instructions:

1. Blend the spinach, banana, avocado, almond milk, and flax seeds until smooth.

2. Pour the smoothie into a bowl.

3. Add your favourite toppings, such as kiwi slices, shredded coconut and pumpkin seeds.

4. Serve immediately and enjoy!

Overnight Oats

Overnight oats are a convenient and nutritious breakfast option. Prepare them the night before, and they'll be ready to eat in the morning.

Classic Overnight Oats Ingredients:
- 1/2 cup rolled oats
- 1/2 cup unsweetened almond milk
- 1/4 cup Greek yogurt
- 1 tablespoon chia seeds
- 1 teaspoon honey or maple syrup
- Toppings: fresh berries, sliced almonds, a drizzle of honey

Instructions:

1. In a jar or bowl, combine the oats, almond milk, Greek yogurt, chia seeds, and honey. Stir well.
2. Cover and refrigerate overnight.
3. In the morning, stir the oats and add your favourite toppings, such as
   fresh berries, sliced almonds, and a drizzle of honey.
4. Serve and enjoy!

Chocolate Peanut Butter Overnight Oats Ingredients:
- 1/2 cup rolled oats
- 1/2 cup unsweetened almond milk
- 2 tablespoons peanut butter
- 1 tablespoon cocoa powder
- 1 teaspoon honey or maple syrup
- Toppings: banana slices, dark chocolate chips

Instructions:

1. In a jar or bowl, combine the oats, almond milk, peanut butter, cocoa powder, and honey. Stir well.
2. Cover and refrigerate overnight.
3. In the morning, stir the oats and add your favourite toppings, such as
   banana slices and dark chocolate chips.
4. Serve and enjoy!

Low-Calorie Pancakes
These pancakes are fluffy, delicious, and lower in calories than traditional pancakes.

Banana Oat Pancakes Ingredients:
- 1 cup rolled oats
- 1 banana
- 2 eggs
- 1/4 cup unsweetened almond milk
- 1 teaspoon baking powder
- 1 teaspoon vanilla extract
- Cooking spray or a small amount of coconut oil

Instructions:
1. Blend the oats until they form a fine flour.
2. Add the banana, eggs, almond milk, baking powder, and vanilla extract to the blender. Blend until smooth.
3. Heat a non-stick skillet over medium heat and lightly coat with cooking spray or coconut oil.
4. Pour small amounts of batter onto the skillet to form pancakes.
5. Cook until bubbles form on the surface, then flip and cook until golden brown.
6. Serve with fresh fruit or a small drizzle of maple syrup.

Blueberry Protein Pancakes Ingredients:
• 1 cup rolled oats
• 1/2 cup cottage cheese
• 1/2 cup egg whites (about 4 large egg whites)
• 1/4 cup unsweetened almond milk
• 1 teaspoon baking powder
• 1 teaspoon vanilla extract
• 1/2 cup fresh or frozen blueberries
• Cooking spray or a small amount of coconut oil

Instructions:
1. Blend the oats until they form a fine flour.
2. Add the cottage cheese, egg whites, almond milk, baking powder, and vanilla extract to the blender. Blend until smooth.
3. Gently fold in the blueberries.
4. Heat a non-stick skillet over medium heat and lightly coat with cooking spray or coconut oil.
5. Pour small amounts of batter onto the skillet to form pancakes.
6. Cook until bubbles form on the surface, then flip and cook until golden brown.
7. Serve with additional fresh blueberries and a small drizzle of maple syrup.

Healthy Breakfast Burritos
These breakfast burritos are packed with protein and veggies, making them a perfect low-calorie breakfast option.

Veggie Breakfast Burrito Ingredients:

• 4 large eggs
• 1/4 cup skim milk
• 1/2 cup diced bell peppers
• 1/2 cup diced tomatoes
• 1/4 cup chopped spinach
• 1/4 cup shredded low-fat cheese
• 4 whole wheat tortillas
• Salt and pepper to taste
• Cooking spray

Instructions:
1. In a bowl, whisk the eggs and milk together. Season with salt and pepper.
2. Heat a non-stick skillet over medium heat and lightly coat with cooking spray.
3. Add the bell peppers, tomatoes, and spinach to the skillet. Sauté until the vegetables are tender.
4. Pour the egg mixture into the skillet and scramble until cooked through.
5. Warm the tortillas in the microwave or on a stovetop.
6. Divide the scrambled eggs and vegetables among the tortillas.
7. Sprinkle with shredded cheese and roll up the tortillas to form burritos.
8. Serve immediately or wrap in foil for a grab-and-go breakfast.

Turkey Sausage Breakfast Burrito Ingredients:
• 4 large eggs
• 1/4 cup skim milk
• 1/2 cup cooked turkey sausage crumbles
• 1/4 cup diced onions
• 1/4 cup diced bell peppers
• 1/4 cup shredded low-fat cheese
• 4 whole wheat tortillas
• Salt and pepper to taste
• Cooking spray

Instructions:

1. In a bowl, whisk the eggs and milk together. Season with salt and pepper.
2. Heat a non-stick skillet over medium heat and lightly coat with cooking spray.
3. Add the onions and bell peppers to the skillet. Sauté until the vegetables are tender.
4. Add the turkey sausage crumbles to the skillet and heat through.
5. Pour the egg mixture into the skillet and scramble until cooked through.
6. Warm the tortillas in the microwave or on a stovetop.
7. Divide the scrambled eggs, sausage, and vegetables among the tortillas.
8. Sprinkle with shredded cheese and roll up the tortillas to form burritos.
9. Serve immediately or wrap in foil for a grab-and-go breakfast.
These breakfast recipes are not only low in calories but also packed with nutrients to help you start your day off right. Enjoy these delicious and healthy options as part of your balanced diet.

Chapter 5: Lunch Recipes

Quinoa Salad
Quinoa salad is a versatile and nutritious option for lunch. It's easy to prepare and can be customized with your favourite vegetables and protein sources.

Mediterranean Quinoa Salad Ingredients:
- 1 cup quinoa, rinsed
- 2 cups water or vegetable broth
- 1 cup cherry tomatoes, halved
- 1 cucumber, diced
- 1/2 red onion, finely chopped
- 1/4 cup Kalamata olives, pitted and sliced
- 1/4 cup crumbled feta cheese
- 1/4 cup chopped fresh parsley
- 1/4 cup extra-virgin olive oil
- 2 tablespoons lemon juice
- 1 teaspoon dried oregano
- Salt and pepper to taste

Instructions:
1. In a medium saucepan, bring the quinoa and water (or vegetable broth) to a boil. Reduce heat to low, cover, and simmer for about 15 minutes, or until the quinoa is cooked and the liquid is absorbed. Fluff with a fork and let cool.
2. In a large bowl, combine the cooked quinoa, cherry tomatoes, cucumber, red onion, Kalamata olives, feta cheese, and parsley.
3. In a small bowl, whisk together the olive oil, lemon juice, dried oregano, salt, and pepper.
4. Pour the dressing over the quinoa mixture and toss to combine.
5. Serve immediately or refrigerate for a few hours to allow the flavours to meld.

Southwest Quinoa Salad Ingredients:

1 cup quinoa, rinsed
2 cups water or vegetable broth
1 cup black beans, drained and rinsed
1 cup corn kernels (fresh or frozen)
1 red bell pepper, diced
- 1/2 red onion, finely chopped 1 avocado, diced
- 1/4 cup chopped fresh cilantro
- 1/4 cup lime juice
- 2 tablespoons extra-virgin olive oil
- 1 teaspoon ground cumin
- 1/2 teaspoon chili powder
- Salt and pepper to taste

Instructions:
1. In a medium saucepan, bring the quinoa and water (or vegetable broth) to a boil. Reduce heat to low, cover, and simmer for about 15 minutes, or until the quinoa is cooked and the liquid is absorbed. Fluff with a fork and let cool.
2. In a large bowl, combine the cooked quinoa, black beans, corn, red bell pepper, red onion, avocado, and cilantro.
3. In a small bowl, whisk together the lime juice, olive oil, ground cumin, chili powder, salt, and pepper.
4. Pour the dressing over the quinoa mixture and toss to combine.
5. Serve immediately or refrigerate for a few hours to allow the flavours to meld.

Grilled Chicken Wraps

Grilled chicken wraps are a light and satisfying lunch option. They're easy to prepare and can be customized with your favourite vegetables and sauces.

Greek Chicken Wrap Ingredients:
• 2 boneless, skinless chicken breasts
• 1 tablespoon olive oil
• 1 teaspoon dried oregano
• Salt and pepper to taste
• 4 whole wheat tortillas
• 1 cup mixed greens
• 1/2 cup cherry tomatoes, halved
• 1/2 cucumber, sliced
• 1/4 red onion, thinly sliced
• 1/4 cup crumbled feta cheese
• 1/4 cup tzatziki sauce

Instructions:
1. Preheat the grill to medium-high heat.
2. Brush the chicken breasts with olive oil and season with dried oregano, salt, and pepper.
3. Grill the chicken for about 6-8 minutes per side, or until fully cooked. Let the chicken rest for a few minutes, then slice into strips.
4. Warm the tortillas on the grill or in a microwave.
5. To assemble the wraps, place a handful of mixed greens on each tortilla, then top with grilled chicken strips, cherry tomatoes, cucumber slices, red onion, feta cheese, and a spoonful of tzatziki sauce.
6. Roll up the tortillas and serve immediately.

Asian Chicken Wrap Ingredients:
• 2 boneless, skinless chicken breasts
• 1 tablespoon soy sauce
• 1 tablespoon hoisin sauce
• 1 teaspoon sesame oil
• 4 whole wheat tortillas
• 1 cup shredded cabbage
• 1/2 cup shredded carrots
• 1/2 red bell pepper, thinly sliced
• 1/4 cup chopped fresh cilantro
• 2 tablespoons chopped peanuts (optional)
• 2 tablespoons peanut sauce (optional)

Instructions:
1. Preheat the grill to medium-high heat.

2. In a small bowl, mix together the soy sauce, hoisin sauce, and sesame oil. Brush the chicken breasts with the sauce mixture.

3. Grill the chicken for about 6-8 minutes per side, or until fully cooked. Let the chicken rest for a few minutes, then slice into strips.

4. Warm the tortillas on the grill or in a microwave.

5. To assemble the wraps, place a handful of shredded cabbage on each tortilla, then top with grilled chicken strips, shredded carrots, red bell pepper slices, cilantro, chopped peanuts, and a drizzle of peanut sauce.

6. Roll up the tortillas and serve immediately.

Veggie Stir-Fry

Veggie stir-fry is a quick and healthy lunch option that can be made with your favourite vegetables and a simple sauce.

Classic Veggie Stir-Fry Ingredients:

- 1 tablespoon olive oil or sesame oil
- 2 cloves garlic, minced
- 1-inch piece of ginger, grated
- 1 red bell pepper, sliced
- 1 yellow bell pepper, sliced
- 1 cup broccoli florets
- 1 cup snap peas
- 1 cup sliced mushrooms
- 1 carrot, thinly sliced
- 1/4 cup soy sauce
- 1 tablespoon hoisin sauce
- 1 tablespoon rice vinegar
- 1 teaspoon sesame seeds (optional)
- Cooked brown rice or quinoa for serving

Instructions:

1. Heat the oil in a large skillet or wok over medium-high heat.

2. Add the garlic and ginger and sauté for 1-2 minutes until fragrant.

3. Add the bell peppers, broccoli, snap peas, mushrooms, and carrot to the skillet. Stir-fry for about 5-7 minutes, or until the vegetables are tender-crisp.

4. In a small bowl, mix together the soy sauce, hoisin sauce, and rice vinegar. Pour the sauce over the vegetables and stir to coat.

5. Cook for another 2-3 minutes until the sauce is heated through.

6. Serve the stir-fry over cooked brown rice or quinoa and sprinkle with sesame seeds if desired.

Tofu Veggie Stir-Fry Ingredients:
• 1 tablespoon olive oil or sesame oil
• 2 cloves garlic, minced
• 1-inch piece of ginger, grated
• 1 block firm tofu, drained and cubed
• 1 red bell pepper, sliced
• 1 cup broccoli florets
• 1 cup snap peas
• 1/2 cup sliced water chestnuts
• 1 carrot, thinly sliced
• 1/4 cup soy sauce
• 1 tablespoon hoisin sauce
• 1 tablespoon rice vinegar
• 1 teaspoon sesame seeds (optional)
• Cooked brown rice or quinoa for serving

Instructions:
1. Heat the oil in a large skillet or wok over medium-high heat.
2. Add the garlic and ginger and sauté for 1-2 minutes until fragrant.
3. Add the tofu cubes to the skillet and cook for about 5 minutes, turning occasionally, until golden brown.
4. Add the bell pepper, broccoli, snap peas, water chestnuts, and carrot to the skillet. Stir-fry for about 5-7 minutes, or until the vegetables are tender-crisp.
5. In a small bowl, mix together the soy sauce, hoisin sauce, and rice vinegar. Pour the sauce over the tofu and vegetables and stir to coat.
6. Cook for another 2-3 minutes until the sauce is heated through.
7. Serve the stir-fry over cooked brown rice or quinoa and sprinkle with sesame seeds if desired.

Low-Calorie Soups
Soups are a comforting and filling lunch option. They can be made ahead of time and stored for quick and easy meals.

Vegetable Soup Ingredients:
- 1 tablespoon olive oil
- 1 onion, chopped
- 2 cloves garlic, minced
- 2 carrots, sliced
- 2 celery stalks, sliced
- 1 zucchini, diced
- 1 cup green beans, trimmed and cut into 1-inch pieces
- 1 can (14.5 ounces) diced tomatoes
- 6 cups vegetable broth
- 1 teaspoon dried basil
- 1 teaspoon dried oregano
- 1/2 teaspoon dried thyme
- Salt and pepper to taste
- 2 cups chopped kale or spinach

Instructions:
1. Heat the olive oil in a large pot over medium heat.
2. Add the onion and garlic and sauté for about 5 minutes, until the onion is translucent.
3. Add the carrots, celery, zucchini, and green beans. Cook for another 5 minutes, stirring occasionally.
4. Add the diced tomatoes, vegetable broth, basil, oregano, thyme, salt, and pepper. Bring to a boil, then reduce heat and simmer for 20-25 minutes, until the vegetables are tender.
5. Stir in the kale or spinach and cook for another 5 minutes, until wilted.
6. Serve hot and enjoy!

Lentil Soup Ingredients:
- 1 tablespoon olive oil
- 1 onion, chopped
- 2 cloves garlic, minced
- 2 carrots, sliced
- 2 celery stalks, sliced
- 1 cup dried lentils, rinsed
- 1 can (14.5 ounces) diced tomatoes
- 6 cups vegetable broth
- 1 teaspoon ground cumin
- 1/2 teaspoon ground coriander
- 1/2 teaspoon ground turmeric
- Salt and pepper to taste
- 2 cups chopped spinach or kale

Instructions:
1. Heat the olive oil in a large pot over medium heat.
2. Add the onion and garlic and sauté for about 5 minutes, until the onion is translucent.
3. Add the carrots and celery and cook for another 5 minutes, stirring occasionally.
4. Add the lentils, diced tomatoes, vegetable broth, cumin, coriander, turmeric, salt, and pepper. Bring to a boil, then reduce heat and simmer for 30-35 minutes, until the lentils are tender.
5. Stir in the spinach or kale and cook for another 5 minutes, until wilted.
6. Serve hot and enjoy!

These lunch recipes are delicious, nutritious, and perfect for keeping your calorie intake in check. Enjoy these healthy options as part of your balanced diet.

Chapter 6: Dinner Recipes

Grilled Fish
Grilled fish is a healthy and delicious option for dinner. It's low in calories and high in protein and healthy fats.
Lemon Herb Grilled SalmonIngredients:
- 4 salmon fillets
- 2 tablespoons olive oil
- 2 tablespoons lemon juice
- 1 tablespoon chopped fresh dill
- 1 tablespoon chopped fresh parsley
- 2 cloves garlic, minced
- Salt and pepper to taste
- Lemon wedges for serving

Instructions:
1. Preheat the grill to medium-high heat.
2. In a small bowl, whisk together the olive oil, lemon juice, dill, parsley, garlic, salt, and pepper.
3. Brush the salmon fillets with the olive oil mixture.
4. Grill the salmon for about 4-5 minutes per side, or until fully cooked.
5. Serve with lemon wedges and your favourite grilled vegetables.

Cilantro Lime Grilled Tilapia Ingredients:
• 4 tilapia fillets
• 2 tablespoons olive oil
• 2 tablespoons lime juice
  • 1 tablespoon chopped fresh cilantro
  • 2 cloves garlic, minced
  • Salt and pepper to taste
  • Lime wedges for serving

Instructions:
1. Preheat the grill to medium-high heat.
2. In a small bowl, whisk together the olive oil, lime juice, cilantro, garlic, salt, and pepper.
3. Brush the tilapia fillets with the olive oil mixture.
4. Grill the tilapia for about 3-4 minutes per side, or until fully cooked.
5. Serve with lime wedges and your favourite grilled vegetables.

Stir-Fried Vegetables with Tofu
Stir-fried vegetables with tofu is a quick and easy dinner option that is both nutritious and satisfying.

Ingredients:
  • 1 tablespoon sesame oil
  • 2 cloves garlic, minced
  • 1-inch piece of ginger, grated
  • 1 block firm tofu, drained and cubed
  • 1 red bell pepper, sliced
  • 1 yellow bell pepper, sliced
  • 1 cup broccoli florets
  • 1 cup snap peas
  • 1/2 cup sliced mushrooms
  • 1 carrot, thinly sliced
  • 1/4 cup soy sauce
  • 1 tablespoon hoisin sauce
  • 1 tablespoon rice vinegar
  • 1 teaspoon sesame seeds (optional)

• Cooked brown rice or quinoa for serving

Instructions:

1. Heat the sesame oil in a large skillet or wok over medium-high heat.
2. Add the garlic and ginger and sauté for 1-2 minutes until fragran†
3. Add the tofu cubes to the skillet and cook for about 5 minutes, turning occasionally, until golden brown.
4. Add the bell peppers, broccoli, snap peas, mushrooms, and carro to the skillet. Stir-fry for about 5-7 minutes, or until the vegetables are tender-crisp.
5. In a small bowl, mix together the soy sauce, hoisin sauce, and rice vinegar. Pour the sauce over the tofu and vegetables and stir to coat.
6. Cook for another 2-3 minutes until the sauce is heated through.
7. Serve the stir-fry over cooked brown rice or quinoa and sprinkle with sesame seeds if desired.

Baked Chicken Breast

Baked chicken breast is a versatile and easy-to-make dinner option It can be paired with a variety of side dishes for a complete meal.

Herb Baked Chicken Breast Ingredients:

- 4 boneless, skinless chicken breasts
- 2 tablespoons olive oil
- 1 tablespoon chopped fresh rosemary
- 1 tablespoon chopped fresh thyme
- 2 cloves garlic, minced
- Salt and pepper to taste
- Lemon wedges for serving

Instructions:

1. Preheat the oven to 375°F (190°C).
2. In a small bowl, mix together the olive oil, rosemary, thyme, garlic, salt, and pepper.
3. Brush the chicken breasts with the olive oil mixture.
4. Place the chicken breasts in a baking dish and bake for about 25-30 minutes, or until fully cooked.
5. Serve with lemon wedges and your favourite side dishes.

Garlic Parmesan Baked Chicken Breast Ingredients:
• 4 boneless, skinless chicken breasts
• 2 tablespoons olive oil
• 1/4 cup grated Parmesan cheese
• 2 cloves garlic, minced
• 1 teaspoon dried basil
• 1 teaspoon dried oregano
• Salt and pepper to taste

Instructions:
1. Preheat the oven to 375°F (190°C).
2. In a small bowl, mix together the olive oil, Parmesan cheese, garlic, basil, oregano, salt, and pepper.
3. Brush the chicken breasts with the olive oil mixture.
4. Place the chicken breasts in a baking dish and bake for about 25-30 minutes, or until fully cooked.
5. Serve with your favourite side dishes.

Spaghetti Squash

Spaghetti squash is a low-calorie alternative to pasta. It can be paired with a variety of sauces and toppings for a satisfying dinner.

Spaghetti Squash with Marinara Sauce Ingredients:
• 1 large spaghetti squash
• 2 tablespoons olive oil
• 1 onion, chopped
• 2 cloves garlic, minced

- 1 can (28 ounces) crushed tomatoes
- 1 teaspoon dried basil
- 1 teaspoon dried oregano
- Salt and pepper to taste
- Fresh basil leaves for garnish

Instructions:

1. Preheat the oven to 400°F (200°C).
2. Cut the spaghetti squash in half lengthwise and scoop out the seeds.
3. Place the squash halves cut-side down on a baking sheet and bake for about 40-45 minutes, or until the flesh is tender.
4. While the squash is baking, heat the olive oil in a large skillet over medium heat.
5. Add the onion and garlic and sauté for about 5 minutes, until the onion is translucent.
6. Add the crushed tomatoes, basil, oregano, salt, and pepper. Simmer for about 20 minutes, stirring occasionally.
7. When the squash is done, use a fork to scrape the flesh into spaghetti-like strands.
8. Serve the spaghetti squash topped with marinara sauce and fresh basil leaves.

Spaghetti Squash with Pesto and Cherry Tomatoes Ingredients:

- 1 large spaghetti squash
- 2 tablespoons olive oil
- 1 cup cherry tomatoes, halved
- 1/4 cup pesto sauce
- 1/4 cup grated Parmesan cheese
- Salt and pepper to taste
- Fresh basil leaves for garnish

Instructions:

1. Preheat the oven to 400°F (200°C).
2. Cut the spaghetti squash in half lengthwise and scoop out the seeds.
3. Place the squash halves cut-side down on a baking sheet and bake for about 40-45 minutes, or until the flesh is tender.
4. While the squash is baking, heat the olive oil in a large skillet over medium heat.
5. Add the cherry tomatoes and cook for about 5 minutes, until they begin to soften.

6. When the squash is done, use a fork to scrape the flesh into spaghetti-like strands.
7. In a large bowl, toss the spaghetti squash with the cooked cherry tomatoes, pesto sauce, and Parmesan cheese. Season with salt and pepper to taste.
8. Serve garnished with fresh basil leaves.
Stuffed Bell Peppers
Stuffed bell peppers are a colourful and nutritious dinner option. They can be filled with a variety of ingredients to suit your taste.

Quinoa and Black Bean Stuffed Peppers Ingredients:
- 4 large bell peppers (any colour)
- 1 tablespoon olive oil
- 1 onion, chopped
- 2 cloves garlic, minced
- 1 cup cooked quinoa
- 1 can (15 ounces) black beans, drained and rinsed
- 1 cup corn kernels (fresh or frozen)
- 1 cup diced tomatoes
- 1 teaspoon ground cumin
- 1/2 teaspoon chili powder
- Salt and pepper to taste
- 1/4 cup shredded low-fat cheese (optional)

Instructions:
1. Preheat the oven to 375°F (190°C).
2. Cut the tops off the bell peppers and remove the seeds and membranes.
3. In a large skillet, heat the olive oil over medium heat.
4. Add the onion and garlic and sauté for about 5 minutes, until the onion is translucent.
5. Stir in the cooked quinoa, black beans, corn, diced tomatoes, cumin, chili powder, salt, and pepper. Cook for another 5 minutes, until heated through.
6. Stuff the bell peppers with the quinoa mixture and place them in a baking dish.
7. If using cheese, sprinkle a little on top of each stuffed pepper.
8. Cover the baking dish with foil and bake for about 25-30 minutes. Remove the foil and bake for another 5-10 minutes, until the peppers are tender and the cheese is melted.
9. Serve hot and enjoy!

Turkey and Spinach Stuffed Peppers Ingredients:
• 4 large bell peppers (any colour)
• 1 tablespoon olive oil
• 1 onion, chopped
• 2 cloves garlic, minced
• 1 pound ground turkey
• 2 cups fresh spinach, chopped
• 1 cup cooked brown rice
• 1 can (15 ounces) diced tomatoes
• 1 teaspoon dried oregano
• 1 teaspoon dried basil
• Salt and pepper to taste
• 1/4 cup shredded low-fat cheese (optional)
Instructions:
1. Preheat the oven to 375°F (190°C).
2. Cut the tops off the bell peppers and remove the seeds and membranes.
3. In a large skillet, heat the olive oil over medium heat.
4. Add the onion and garlic and sauté for about 5 minutes, until the onion is translucent.
5. Add the ground turkey and cook for about 7-10 minutes, until browned and fully cooked.
6. Stir in the chopped spinach, cooked brown rice, diced tomatoes, oregano, basil, salt, and pepper. Cook for another 5 minutes, until heated through.
7. Stuff the bell peppers with the turkey mixture and place them in a baking dish.
8. If using cheese, sprinkle a little on top of each stuffed pepper.
9. Cover the baking dish with foil and bake for about 25-30 minutes. Remove the foil and bake for another 5-10 minutes, until the peppers are tender and the cheese is melted.
10. Serve hot and enjoy!

These dinner recipes are designed to be healthy, delicious, and satisfying, perfect for ending your day on a nutritious note. Enjoy the low-calorie options as part of your healthy living journey.

Chapter 7: Snacks and Sides

Healthy Snacks

Snacking can be a part of a healthy diet if you choose nutrient-dense, low-calorie options. Here are some ideas for healthy snacks that are both delicious and satisfying.

Apple Slices with Almond Butter Ingredients:

• 1 apple, sliced

• 2 tablespoons almond butter

Instructions:

1. Wash and slice the apple into thin wedges.

2. Serve with a side of almond butter for dipping.

Greek Yogurt with Berries Ingredients:

• 1 cup Greek yogurt

• 1/2 cup mixed berries (blueberries, strawberries, raspberries)

• 1 teaspoon honey (optional)

• 1 tablespoon chopped nuts (optional)

Instructions:

1. Spoon the Greek yogurt into a bowl.

2. Top with mixed berries.

3. Drizzle with honey and sprinkle with chopped nuts if desired.

Hummus and Veggie Sticks Ingredients:

• 1 cup hummus

• 1 carrot, cut into sticks

• 1 cucumber, cut into sticks

• 1 red bell pepper, cut into sticks

• 1 celery stalk, cut into sticks

Instructions:

1. Arrange the veggie sticks on a plate.

2. Serve with a side of hummus for dipping.

Roasted Chickpeas Ingredients:

• 1 can (15 ounces) chickpeas, drained and rinsed

• 1 tablespoon olive oil

• 1 teaspoon smoked paprika

• 1/2 teaspoon garlic powder

• 1/2 teaspoon onion powder

• Salt and pepper to taste

Instructions:
1. Preheat the oven to 400°F (200°C).
2. Pat the chickpeas dry with a paper towel.
3. In a bowl, toss the chickpeas with olive oil, smoked paprika, garlic powder, onion powder, salt, and pepper.
4. Spread the chickpeas on a baking sheet in a single layer.
5. Roast for 20-30 minutes, stirring halfway through, until crispy.
6. Let cool and enjoy as a crunchy snack.

Nutritious Sides

These sides are perfect complements to your main dishes. They are nutritious, low in calories, and add a burst of flavour to your meals.

Garlic Roasted Brussels Sprouts Ingredients:
• 1 pound Brussels sprouts, trimmed and halved
• 2 tablespoons olive oil
• 2 cloves garlic, minced
• Salt and pepper to taste
• 1 tablespoon balsamic vinegar (optional)

Instructions:
1. Preheat the oven to 400°F (200°C).
2. In a large bowl, toss the Brussels sprouts with olive oil, garlic, salt, and pepper.
3. Spread the Brussels sprouts on a baking sheet in a single layer.
4. Roast for 20-25 minutes, stirring halfway through, until golden brown and crispy.
5. Drizzle with balsamic vinegar if desired before serving.

Quinoa and Kale Salad Ingredients:
• 1 cup quinoa, rinsed
• 2 cups water or vegetable broth
• 2 cups chopped kale
• 1/4 cup chopped red onion
• 1/4 cup dried cranberries
• 1/4 cup crumbled feta cheese
• 2 tablespoons olive oil
• 2 tablespoons lemon juice
• Salt and pepper to taste

Instructions:
1. In a medium saucepan, bring the quinoa and water (or vegetable broth) to a boil. Reduce heat to low, cover, and simmer for about 15 minutes, or until the quinoa is cooked and the liquid is absorbed. Fluff with a fork and let cool.
2. In a large bowl, combine the cooked quinoa, chopped kale, red onion, dried cranberries, and feta cheese.
3. In a small bowl, whisk together the olive oil, lemon juice, salt, and pepper.
4. Pour the dressing over the quinoa mixture and toss to combine.
5. Serve immediately or refrigerate for a few hours to allow the flavours to meld.

Sweet Potato Fries Ingredients:
- 2 large sweet potatoes, peeled and cut into fries
- 2 tablespoons olive oil
- 1 teaspoon smoked paprika
- 1/2 teaspoon garlic powder
- 1/2 teaspoon salt
- 1/4 teaspoon black pepper

Instructions:
1. Preheat the oven to 425°F (220°C).
2. In a large bowl, toss the sweet potato fries with olive oil, smoked paprika, garlic powder, salt, and pepper.
3. Spread the sweet potato fries on a baking sheet in a single layer.
4. Bake for 25-30 minutes, turning halfway through, until crispy and golden brown.
5. Serve hot and enjoy!

Cucumber and Tomato Salad Ingredients:
• 2 cucumbers, sliced
• 1 pint cherry tomatoes, halved
• 1/4 red onion, thinly sliced
• 1/4 cup chopped fresh parsley
• 2 tablespoons olive oil
• 2 tablespoons red wine vinegar
• Salt and pepper to taste
Instructions:
1. In a large bowl, combine the cucumbers, cherry tomatoes, red onion, and parsley.
2. In a small bowl, whisk together the olive oil, red wine vinegar, salt, and pepper.
3. Pour the dressing over the cucumber mixture and toss to combine.
4. Serve immediately or refrigerate for a few hours to allow the flavours to meld.

These snacks and sides are perfect for adding variety to your diet while keeping your calorie intake in check. Enjoy these healthy options as part of your balanced eating plan.

Chapter 8: Healthy Desserts

Indulgent yet Low-Calorie Treats

Desserts don't have to be off-limits when you're aiming for a healthy diet. Here are some delicious, low-calorie dessert options that allow you to enjoy a sweet treat without compromising your health goals.
Greek Yogurt with Honey and Nuts Ingredients:
• 1 cup Greek yogurt
• 1 tablespoon honey
• 1 tablespoon chopped nuts (almonds, walnuts, or pistachios)
• 1/2 teaspoon cinnamon (optional)
Instructions:
1. Spoon the Greek yogurt into a serving bowl.
2. Drizzle with honey.
3. Sprinkle with chopped nuts and cinnamon if desired.
4. Serve immediately.

Frozen Banana Bites Ingredients:
• 2 bananas, sliced into rounds
• 1/2 cup dark chocolate chips
• 1 tablespoon coconut oil
• 1/4 cup shredded coconut (optional)
Instructions:
1. Line a baking sheet with parchment paper.
2. Place the banana slices on the baking sheet and freeze for 1 hour.
3. In a microwave-safe bowl, combine the dark chocolate chips and coconut oil. Microwave in 30-second intervals, stirring between each, until the chocolate is melted and smooth.
4. Dip each frozen banana slice into the melted chocolate, then place it back on the baking sheet. Sprinkle with shredded coconut if desired.
5. Freeze for another 30 minutes, or until the chocolate is set.
6. Store in an airtight container in the freezer and enjoy as a frozen treat.

Chia Seed Pudding Ingredients:
• 1/4 cup chia seeds
• 1 cup unsweetened almond milk (or any milk of choice)
• 1 tablespoon maple syrup or honey
• 1/2 teaspoon vanilla extract
• Fresh berries or fruit for topping
Instructions:
1. In a bowl, whisk together the chia seeds, almond milk, maple syrup (or honey), and vanilla extract.
2. Let the mixture sit for about 10 minutes, then whisk again to prevent clumping.
3. Cover and refrigerate for at least 4 hours or overnight, until the pudding has thickened.
4. Stir well before serving and top with fresh berries or fruit.

Baked Apples with Cinnamon Ingredients:
• 4 apples, cored
• 2 tablespoons maple syrup or honey
• 1 teaspoon ground cinnamon
• 1/4 cup chopped nuts (optional)
Instructions:
1. Preheat the oven to 350°F (175°C).
2. Place the apples in a baking dish.
3. Drizzle with maple syrup (or honey) and sprinkle with ground cinnamon.
4. If desired, fill the cores with chopped nuts.
5. Bake for 20-25 minutes, or until the apples are tender.
6. Serve warm, and enjoy!
Avocado Chocolate Mousse Ingredients:
• 2 ripe avocados
• 1/4 cup cocoa powder
• 1/4 cup honey or maple syrup
• 1/4 cup almond milk (or any milk of choice)
• 1 teaspoon vanilla extract
• Fresh berries or nuts for topping (optional)
Instructions:
1. In a blender or food processor, combine the avocados, cocoa powder, honey (or maple syrup), almond milk, and vanilla extract.
2. Blend until smooth and creamy.
3. Taste and adjust sweetness if necessary.
4. Spoon the mousse into serving dishes and chill for at least 1 hour.
5. Top with fresh berries or nuts if desired before serving.
Banana Oat Cookies Ingredients:
• 2 ripe bananas, mashed
• 1 cup rolled oats
• 1/4 cup dark chocolate chips (optional)
• 1/4 cup chopped nuts (optional)
• 1 teaspoon vanilla extract
Instructions:
1. Preheat the oven to 350°F (175°C).
2. In a large bowl, mix together the mashed bananas, rolled oats, dark chocolate chips, chopped nuts, and vanilla extract.
3. Drop spoonful of the dough onto a baking sheet lined with parchment paper.
4. Bake for 12-15 minutes, or until the cookies are golden brown.
5. Let cool on a wire rack before serving.

Berry Smoothie Bowl Ingredients:
• 1 cup frozen mixed berries
• 1 banana
• 1/2 cup Greek yogurt
• 1/2 cup almond milk (or any milk of choice)
• 1 tablespoon honey or maple syrup (optional)
• Toppings: fresh berries, granola, chia seeds, coconut flakes
Instructions:
1. In a blender, combine the frozen mixed berries, banana, Greek yogurt, almond milk, and honey (or maple syrup).
2. Blend until smooth and thick.
3. Pour into a bowl and top with your favourite toppings, such as fresh berries, granola, chia seeds, and coconut flakes.
4. Serve immediately and enjoy!

These healthy dessert recipes are perfect for satisfying your sweet tooth without the guilt. Enjoy these low-calorie treats as part of your balanced diet and healthy living journey.

Chapter 9: Beverages

Refreshing and Healthy Drinks

Staying hydrated is crucial for overall health, and enjoying a variety of beverages can make it easier and more enjoyable. Here are some delicious, low-calorie beverage options to keep you refreshed and hydrated.

Detox Water Ingredients:
- 1 lemon, sliced
- 1 cucumber, sliced
- 1/2 cup fresh mint leaves
- 8 cups water

Instructions:
1. In a large pitcher, combine the lemon slices, cucumber slices, and mint leaves.
2. Fill the pitcher with water.
3. Refrigerate for at least 2 hours to allow the flavours to infuse.
4. Serve chilled and enjoy throughout the day.

Green Smoothie Ingredients:
• 1 cup spinach
• 1/2 cup kale
• 1 banana
• 1/2 cup frozen pineapple
• 1/2 cup frozen mango
• 1 cup coconut water (or any liquid of choice)
Instructions:
1. In a blender, combine the spinach, kale, banana, frozen pineapple, frozen mango, and coconut water.
2. Blend until smooth and creamy.
3. Pour into a glass and enjoy immediately.
Herbal Iced Tea Ingredients:
• 4 cups water
• 4 herbal tea bags (chamomile, peppermint, or your favourite herbal tea)
• 1 tablespoon honey or agave nectar (optional)
• Lemon slices and fresh mint for garnish
Instructions:
1. Bring the water to a boil in a large pot.
2. Remove from heat and add the herbal tea bags.
3. Let steep for about 5-10 minutes, depending on desired strength.
4. Remove the tea bags and stir in honey or agave nectar if using.
5. Let the tea cool to room temperature, then refrigerate until chilled.
6. Serve over ice with lemon slices and fresh mint.

Coconut Water Smoothie Ingredients:
• 1 cup coconut water
• 1/2 cup Greek yogurt
• 1/2 cup frozen berries (strawberries, blueberries, or raspberries)
• 1/2 banana
• 1 tablespoon chia seeds (optional)
Instructions:
1. In a blender, combine the coconut water, Greek yogurt, frozen berries, banana, and chia seeds if using.
2. Blend until smooth and creamy.
3. Pour into a glass and enjoy immediately.

Golden Milk (Turmeric Latte) Ingredients:
• 1 cup unsweetened almond milk (or any milk of choice)
• 1/2 teaspoon ground turmeric
• 1/4 teaspoon ground ginger
• 1/4 teaspoon ground cinnamon
• 1 teaspoon honey or maple syrup (optional)
• Pinch of black pepper

Instructions:
1. In a small saucepan, combine the almond milk, turmeric, ginger, cinnamon, honey (or maple syrup), and black pepper.
2. Heat over medium heat, whisking constantly, until the mixture is hot but not boiling.
3. Pour into a mug and enjoy warm.

Berry Infused Water Ingredients:
• 1/2 cup fresh or frozen berries (strawberries, blueberries, raspberries)
• 1 lime, sliced
• 8 cups water

Instructions:
1. In a large pitcher, combine the berries and lime slices.
2. Fill the pitcher with water.
3. Refrigerate for at least 2 hours to allow the flavours to infuse.
4. Serve chilled and enjoy throughout the day.

Matcha Green Tea Latte Ingredients:
• 1 teaspoon matcha green tea powder
• 1/4 cup hot water
• 3/4 cup unsweetened almond milk (or any milk of choice)
• 1 teaspoon honey or agave nectar (optional)

Instructions:
1. In a small bowl, whisk the matcha green tea powder with the hot water until smooth and frothy.
2. In a small saucepan, heat the almond milk over medium heat until hot but not boiling.
3. Pour the matcha mixture into a mug and stir in the hot almond milk.
4. Sweeten with honey or agave nectar if desired.
5. Enjoy warm or over ice.

Chia Seed Lemonade Ingredients:
• 4 cups water
• 1/4 cup fresh lemon juice (about 2 lemons)
• 2 tablespoons chia seeds
• 1-2 tablespoons honey or agave nectar (optional)
Instructions:
1. In a large pitcher, combine the water, lemon juice, chia seeds, and honey or agave nectar if using.
2. Stir well and let sit for about 10 minutes, stirring occasionally, until the chia seeds begin to swell and gel.
3. Serve over ice and enjoy.
These healthy beverages are perfect for staying hydrated and refreshed while keeping your calorie intake in check. Enjoy these delicious options as part of your healthy living journey.

Conclusion

Embarking on a journey toward healthy living through low-calorie foods is a rewarding and transformative experience. By incorporating the delicious and nutritious recipes in this book, you can enjoy a varie of meals, snacks, beverages, and desserts that support your health ar wellness goals without sacrificing flavour or satisfaction.

Key Takeaways

• **Balanced Nutrition**: Each chapter provides a range of options to ensure you're getting a balanced intake of essential nutrients. From hearty breakfasts and satisfying lunches to energizing snacks and hydrating beverages, these recipes are designed to fuel your body and mind.

• **Flavourful and Satisfying**: Healthy eating doesn't mean bland and boring. The recipes here are packed with flavours', using fresh ingredients and creative combinations to keep your taste buds happy.

• **Sustainable Habits**: Adopting a healthy diet is more than a temporary change; it's about creating sustainable habits that you can maintain in the long run. These recipes are easy to prepare and integrate into your daily routine, making it simpler to stick to your healthy living goals.

• **Mindful Choices**: Choosing low-calorie, nutrient-dense foods helps manage weight and improve overall health. This book encourages mindful eating, where you listen to your body's needs and make choices that nourish and satisfy.

Moving Forward

As you continue on your healthy living journey, remember that consistency and enjoyment are key. Here are a few tips to help you stay on track:

• **Plan Ahead**: Take some time each week to plan your meals and snacks. Having a plan can help you make healthier choices and avoid last-minute temptations.

• **Stay Hydrated:** Drink plenty of water throughout the day. Infused waters and herbal teas are great ways to add variety to your hydration routine.

• **Listen to Your Body**: Pay attention to hunger and fullness cues. Eat when you're hungry, and stop when you're satisfied.

• **Be Flexible**: It's okay to indulge occasionally. Enjoy your favourite treats in moderation and balance them with healthier options.

• **Stay Active**: Combine your healthy eating habits with regular physical activity. Find exercises you enjoy and make them a part of your routine.

Final Thoughts

Healthy living is a continuous journey filled with opportunities to learn and grow. By incorporating these low-calorie, nutrient-rich recipes into your daily life, you're taking a significant step toward a healthier, happier you. Enjoy the process, celebrate your successes, and keep exploring new ways to nourish your body and mind. Here's to your health and wellness! Enjoy every bite, sip, and moment on your journey to a vibrant, balanced life.

References

Academy of Nutrition and Dietetics. (2022). Food & Nutrition Information. Retrieved from https://www.eatright.org

American Heart Association. (2022). Healthy Eating. Retrieved from https://www.heart.org/en/healthy-living

Centres for Disease Control and Prevention. (2022). Healthy Eating for a Healthy Weight. Retrieved from https://www.cdc.gov/healthyweight

Harvard T.H. Chan School of Public Health. (2022). The Nutrition Source. Retrieved from https://www.hsph.harvard.edu/nutritionsource

Mayo Clinic. (2022). Nutrition and Healthy Eating. Retrieved from https://www.mayoclinic.org/healthy-lifestyle

National Institutes of Health. (2022). Healthy Eating Plan. Retrieved from https://www.nih.gov/health-information/healthy-eating

World Health Organization. (2022). Nutrition. Retrieved from https://www.who.int/health-topics/nutrition